Simplifying Nutritional Wealth Series

A series of small, easy to read books addressing common health issues women tend to have through their years. I have decided to mainly deal with WOMEN because we seem to throw hormones into the mix of everyday life. A lot of what we deal with and how we deal with obstacles comes from an emotional view. All we need to do is grab a hold of our hormones, keep them in balance and POOF…problem solved.

If we can understand the dynamics of controlling these hormones with nutrition, women will completely control the world they live in!! ENJOY!!
Isra Girgrah Wynn

I0449515

ISBN: 978-1-312-59236-0

http://www.iwynn.net

Acknowledgements:
Thank you to everyone who supports
my vision, especially my loving
husband, Marty Wynn. And thanks to
my children who keep me on my toes
24/7.

Cravings: Why Do I Want That!!!

A food craving is an intense desire to consume a specific food, and is different from normal hunger. Hunger and cravings are different sensations. The body regulates hunger. Hunger serves more practical purpose signaling our brains that it is time to eat. The mind wields greater power over cravings. There is no single explanation for food cravings, and explanations range from low **serotonin** levels affecting brain centers for appetite to production of **endorphins** as a result of consuming fats and carbohydrates. There are approximately 35 of 70+ chemicals that influence when and what we eat.

As we age, it's all about the sensory memories that we form in relation to food. We only crave the foods that we've had before. Granted, much of what we desire is fattening or high in calories!! How can you crave something you have never had? Our food cravings are physiological ways to seek out familiar pleasures.

Cravings start in the BRAIN. Neurotransmitters, nerve chemicals, send messages from the body to the brain. These neurotransmitters regulate nerve function, including memory, appetite, mental function, mood, movement, and wake-sleep cycle.

Chemicals are released when you eat food, any food, good tasting or not. These chemicals and areas of the brain are the same as those involved in drug response and addiction. Food can act like a drug to the brain. The same chain of events happen; release of chemical, making person feel good, and want to continue that feeling. We learn to need that food to satisfy that craving. The "fast food" joint isn't much different from a person selling "drugs".

So why do people crave items high in fat and calories? Fatty, sugary foods release chemicals called **opioids** into our bloodstream. These opioids bind to receptors in our brains and give us feelings of pleasure and even euphoria. Our bodies, momentarily, give us a thank you for ingesting that box of truffles or whatnot. Our sensory memories of these foods, which elicit that chemical satisfaction, reinforce the cravings.

The body is amazingly efficient. It stores an impression of everything you've ever eaten – every flavor, texture, and chemical make up. If your diet isn't full of a wide variety of nutrients from fruits, vegetables, whole grains, and quality proteins, it will crave the only source it knows of to obtain what it needs…brownies, cookies, chips. And you know why you want to eat the whole bag? Because it takes a larger amount of unhealthy food to give you what your body needs. For example, one serving of butternut squash might supply you with your entire day's need of magnesium but it would take an entire box of chocolate brownies to give you a fraction of the daily requirement. Even flavors of food like salty, sweet, savory, pungent, and sour help your body maintain balance.

A craving is simply the body's way of telling you it needs something…a vitamin, mineral, protein, or nutrient to function properly.

One of the first taps on your shoulder that you get when you have a vitamin, mineral, amino acid, or fatty acid deficiency, is a craving. Recurrent cravings become recurrent taps on your shoulder – clues to pay attention to. Clues to look deeper. Yes, there may be emotional causes, but nutrients are always part of the picture.

Cravings also magnify when we diet, are under stress, skip meals, feel depressed, or are premenstrual. There is a biological connection between changes in body chemicals and food cravings. Food cravings are also fueled by an addiction to pleasure.

What you eat directly and indirectly affects nerve chemicals, which in turn influence your moods and food cravings.

Our food preferences, desires, cravings, and loves are literally hardwired into our basic instincts for survival, safety, and love!

Carbohydrate Cravings
A desire for sweets is hardwired into the brain. Some people crave carbohydrates not because they lack willpower but because they suffer from an imbalance on **serotonin**. In essence, carbohydrate cravers turn to desserts, doughnuts, and other pastries, or even pasta and breads, to relieve dwindling energy levels, hunger, depression, and stress caused by their low serotonin levels. Their carbohydrate-rich snacks raise serotonin levels, curb the craving, and energize them. Cravers are therefore rewarded each time they indulge their cravings, because the food

they eat increases their serotonin levels and makes them feel better.

This carbohydrate-rich meal or snack alters brain chemistry and provides temporary relief from mild depression or tension. Low-carbohydrate weight-loss diets are doomed to fail for these people. Within days of cutting back on carbohydrates, the carbohydrate cravings amplify to the degree that leaves the dieter almost powerless against an all out binge.

Some of the other symptoms of serotonin imbalance are: people who struggle with weight problems, frequently diet, frequently moody or irritable, and likely to drink too much alcohol.

Armies of nerve chemicals are produced by the appetite-control center in the brain, called the **hypothalamus**. When the group of nerve cells that control eating receive messages that fuel stores are threatened (as a consequence of strict dieting or even after a late night fast), they release an array of appetite-

stimulating neurotransmitters, including
neuropeptide Y (NPY), galanin, and the
endorphins, to perk up our desires to
eat.

As NPY levels go up, so do your
cravings for sweets. A quick-weight-loss
diet is likely to send NPY levels soaring,
so don't be surprised after starting such
an eating plan if you are soon battling
uncontrollable food cravings. NPY jump-
starts the eating cycle in the morning.
Sugar stores (glycogen) in the muscles
and liver are drained during the night as
we sleep; waning blood-sugar levels
send a message to release NPY. This
neurotransmitter subtly convinces us to
eat waffles, pancakes, toast, jelly,
doughnuts, and other carbohydrate-rich
foods for breakfast.

Stress also triggers NPY production.

Serotonin and neuropeptide Y (NPY)
are just one piece of the whole picture
when it comes to managing your mood
and carbohydrate cravings. Food
cravings are also fueled by an addiction

to pleasure. Much like the high experienced after doing intense exercise, having a good laugh, or listening to good music, a euphoric or calming response is produced by certain foods that release morphine like chemicals in the brain called **endorphins**. Endorphins make eating tasty, sweet, or creamy foods fun.

While the serotonin & NPY response from eating carbohydrates takes time to elicit, the mere touch of sugar on the tongue produces an immediate endorphin rush. Thus you feel good immediately after eating a doughnut, because of the boost of endorphins, which is followed by a lingering good mood induced by the slow-acting increase in serotonin & NPY.

Endorphins are turned on when we consume sugary snacks, but they also turn on our cravings for sweet-and-creamy foods. Endorphins provide an example of the cyclical manner in which brain chemistry affects eating, which then affects brain chemistry. For example, adopt a low-carbohydrate diet, and the resultant low blood-sugar levels trigger the release of endorphins, which increase our sweet cravings. Lose weight too fast, and fatty acids released from fat tissue also cause an endorphin rush that sends us to the refrigerator in search for a sweet or creamy snack. The sugary snack provides a temporary quick fix, possibly because its effect on endorphins, which worsens cravings in the long run since it strengthens the addiction to these morphine like chemicals.

Eating a sugary diet reduces your chances of consuming enough of the 40+ nutrients you need for your body to function smoothly, and increases losses of minerals essential for normal blood-sugar regulation and the prevention of weight gain.
To boost your mood without jeopardizing your waistline and your health, limit your daily sugar. Further, sidestep your sweet tooth by turning

from highly sugared snacks to minimally processed, wholesome carbohydrates, such as whole grains and starchy vegetables.

Be patient! It will take 2-3 weeks of eating well before your body chemistry will adjust and you notice an improvement in your overall mood and a decrease in your cravings.

While simple carbohydrates such as sugar contribute to the problem, complex, minimally processed carbohydrates are part of the cure. Nutrient packed whole grain breads and cereals, brown rice, and starchy vegetables do not aggravate endorphin levels or blood sugar but they do satisfy serotonin needs. These nutritious foods help curb cravings and soothe moods.

Fat Cravings
Although many people assume they crave sweets and claim they have a sweet tooth, in reality they probably are searching for fat. A desire for fat – or more specifically, sweetened fat – leads some people to indulge in chocolate, ice

cream, and cookies. These so-called carbohydrate-rich foods derive as much, if not more, of their calories from fat than from sugar; the sugar just makes the fat taste better.

Fat alone is unpalatable. Sugar masks the fat in foods. But add even a little sugar and you have a sweet-and-creamy combination that brings out the craving in even the most ardent dieter.

FAT MAKES FOOD DESIRABLE, AND SUGAR MAKES THE FAT INVISIBLE.

The breakdown of body fat, which occurs during dieting or when several hours have passed between meals, releases fat fragments (called free fatty acids) into the blood that travel to the brain and trigger the release of **galanin**.

As galanin levels rise, so does your desire to eat foods that contain fat, such as salad dressing, chocolate, meat, or potato chips. The more galanin you produce, the more fat you eat.

Reproductive hormones such as estrogen, the stress hormone cortisol, elevated insulin and possibly the endorphins also turn on galanin, while dopamine might turn off galanin release.

Galanin is released when fat stores need filling up. In the evening, galanin levels tend to rise, which may be nature's way of making sure that people have enough calories to last them through the night.

Leptin, a hormone that plays a key role in our preferences for fatty foods, regulates body fat. Leptin sends messages to the brain about the body's fat stores. When elevated, it serves as a stop-eating signal by turning off NPY and Galanin but sends a start-eating signal when low by turning on NPY and Galanin. Severe dieting lowers body fat too rapidly, which lowers leptin levels and turns on fat cravings. This might explain why most people inevitably regain the weight they have lost on fad diets.

Leptin also might be influenced by what we eat – in particular, zinc-rich foods. Low zinc intake reduced Leptin levels.

SALT

A craving for something salty is the most elusive of all the urges to eat. No one really knows why some people crave salty potato chips, French fries, salted nuts or popcorn or pizza instead of ice cream or chocolate. Although there is nothing inherently wrong in satisfying a craving for salt, the salty foods that we tend to eat often are major contributors to fat in the diet, which can add unwanted pounds.

One theory for the increased cravings for salty food in women, especially during the two weeks prior to their cycle, could be the effect of the female hormone estrogen on the antidiuretic hormones, vasopressin and aldosterone, which cause fluid retention. Some women gain up to ten pounds of added water weight during this time of the month, which turns on their salt cravings to help maintain the normal salt concentration in the body. Salt cravings could stem from low calcium intake as well. People with low calcium intakes also are most prone to cravings for salty foods. Salt cravings might result from the body's memory of very early experiences. We know the taste for salt is innately appealing to people. However, most people consume much more than they need, which means at least a portion of our salt cravings is habit.

STRESS
To be alive is to be under stress!! Everything from the ring of a doorbell to the loss of a loved one can trigger the stress. Stress is one of those survival of the species basic instincts which meant "fight or flight". Stress is a major player in mood, food cravings, thinking, insomnia, and all aspects of emotional and physical health.
The body releases the hormone **Cortisol** in stressful situations.
The stress hormone Cortisol scrambles our appetite-control chemicals, which

affects food intake and mood. Cortisol reduces the brain's ability to use glucose, especially the hippocampus, which is a relay station for short-term memory. Cortisol turns on the production of Neuropeptide Y (NPY), alters dopamine levels, and lowers serotonin. It's no wonder we make poor food choices when we're stressed, turning to sweets, salty snacks, and processed grains. Consequently, weight gain during stressful times might be a result of this altered chemistry, which prompts overeating, especially sugary foods.

PMS

PMS triggers food cravings. One out of every three women experiences increased hunger and food cravings during the two weeks before her cycle and can consume up to 87 percent more calories than at any other time during the month. A woman's cycle lowers her serotonin levels, which accounts for the mood swings and food cravings. PMS and sweets go hand in hand. Women who are depressed and battle food cravings during premenstrual phase also are most likely to turn to chocolate and other sweets, with sugar increasing by up to 20 teaspoons daily. The most frequent symptoms of PMS including cravings for carbohydrates-rich foods, sleep disturbances, and depression, coincide with dwindling serotonin levels. Low levels of endorphins also might influence PMS symptoms. A surge in the pleasure-producing endorphins coincides with ovulation, but levels drop off during the premenstrual phase, possibly contributing to the depression, hunger, irritability, food cravings, and other mood changes associated with PMS. Eating sweets only aggravates PMS, intensifying the emotional highs and lows, escalating a minor food craving into a binge, and magnifying PMS symptoms.

Perhaps the ultimate hormonal surge, pregnancy can send a woman's food cravings into overdrive. A pregnant woman's sense of taste and smell becomes more acute. Her cravings focus more on intensely sweet, salty, or spicy foods.

Among the more strange food cravings is the phenomenon called **PICA**, which is more prevalent among children and pregnant women. Pica, a physiological eating disorder characterized by the desire to eat nonfood items. Some experiencing pica eat ice and some eat dirt, clay or cornstarch. This type of pica frequently relates to iron deficiencies in pregnant women. Anemic people also have a higher likelihood of encountering pica.

Dieting & Skipping Meals
Limiting your caloric intake through dieting can be tricky business because your body naturally generates more Ghrelin, the hunger hormone, when it thinks you're in danger of starvation. That kick-starts your appetite, which can then open up a Pandora's box of cravings. The pendulum swings from restraint/abstinence to binge, sometimes

resulting in obsessive eating, fear of food, desperation, and anger. The more dieters fail at dieting, the more likely they are to struggle with emotional eating.

Late night cravings for sweet-and-creamy or salty-and-greasy foods are most common when you skip meals, or snack during the day, avoid eating breakfast, or eat too many sugary foods throughout the day. These cravings are a conditioned response; the more often you snack at night, the stronger your body's cravings will be in the future. One out of every four people start every day without breakfast; 50 percent eat breakfast only occasionally. Today, cutting calories to lose weight is one of the main reasons people skip the first meal of the day, along with not having enough time for a meal and not feeling like eating. **Breakfast is the most important meal**. This is the only time during the day that eight, and perhaps ten or more, hours have gone by between meals. The body still needs fuel to keep its millions of metabolic processes functioning.

Levels of neuropeptide Y (NPY) are highest in the morning and jump-start the day's eating cycle by dictating a preference for carbohydrates. NPY is a nerve chemical that ensures we replenish the fuel stores depleted since dinner, so its no wonder breakfast foods are typically high-carbohydrate ones, such as waffles, toast, pancakes, oatmeal, cereal, and fruit. NPY is a very powerful nerve chemical. It doesn't go away just because you skip breakfast. Instead, NPY levels remain on until the cravings lead to overeating later in the day.

Stress adds to the problem, since it amplifies NPY levels. Skip breakfast, then venture into a day filled with time demands, deadlines at work, overbooked schedules, even boredom, and raging NPY levels are boosted even higher by the stress hormones **norepinephrine** (a cousin to adrenalin) and **corticosterone**, both secreted from the adrenal glands. The result is, a day without breakfast can lead to an even greater likelihood of increased food cravings, overeating, and weight gain.

Listen to your cravings. They are telling you something. In many cases, cravings for sweets are an unconscious effort to raise serotonin or NPY levels; a desire for creamy or fatty foods, from ice cream to steak, might be a basic need to satisfy galanin levels. These appetite-control chemicals are very powerful, and trying to use willpower to make them go away is, in many cases, like trying to give up breathing. So work with them instead.

APPENDIX A

Certain foods and lifestyle patterns affect powerful mood-modifying brain chemicals called neurotransmitters.

Serotonin – this is a chemical released after eating carbohydrates (sugar and starches). It enhances calmness, improves mood, and lessens depression. High levels of serotonin help control appetite, satisfy cravings, and provide a feeling of wellbeing and inner calm.

Dopamine and norepinephrine – these are chemicals released after eating protein (meats, poultry, dairy, legumes). They enhance mental concentration and alertness.

Ghrelin – a neurotransmitter that sets up an irresistible urge to eat when elevated.

NPY, neuropeptide Y – increases carbohydrate cravings when elevated

Galanin – increases the desire for fatty foods when elevated

Cortisol – the emergency gland of the body, the adrenals release cortisol as the primary coordinator for the reactions of stress. Cortisol decreases the production of serotonin. If you normally eat to relieve stress, the hormone cortisol places the extra calories (fat) in the abdomen or stomach area of your body.

Endorphins – the body's natural "high" which gives pain relief and pleasure when elevated

APPENDIX B

How does lifestyle and food choices affect your brain chemistry?

As you lower calories to lose weight, you starve your brain first and that depletes serotonin (chemical that helps you feel calm, peaceful, and content, and has a pivotal role in regulating appetite). **This leads to increased cravings** for different foods, depression, anxiety, lethargy, feelings of hopelessness or rage all increase. **Typical dieting** means an immediate cutback on the production of chemicals that support health of your mind, your psyche, and your spirit.

If you skip meals, this will lead to your blood sugar levels going abnormally low and intense cravings start. This also causes an increase in Ghrelin (a chemical that sets up an irresistible urge to eat) and also lowers Neuropeptide Y, which increases carbohydrate cravings.

This will lead to an unstoppable desire to eat lots of food and increases your eating frequency, which leads to binging on extra foods.

As you lower calories to lose weight, this will lower insulin and thyroid hormone, which lowers your metabolism and also lowers the release of fat from your body (you can't lose weight as easily and may end up on a plateau). **As you eat more dietary fat**, this will increase Endorphins (the body's natural "high", which gives pain relief and pleasure). The more fat in a person's diet, the more Galanin (increases the desire for fatty foods) is produced and the more Galanin that's produced, the more one prefers or craves fattier foods. Eating less fat for several weeks reduces Galanin levels and the desire to eat faty foods. **So the less fat (and refined carbohydrates you eat), the less you want.**

Eat only sugar or sweets: Blood sugar quickly (within 10-15 minutes) rises to above-normal levels, followed within 25-

40 minutes by a dramatic drop in blood sugar to subnormal levels.

Eat only refined starches: Blood-sugar levels rise less quickly than sugar but still can rise too high, resulting in too much insulin released from the pancreas and a drop in blood sugar to subnormal levels, but not as dramatic as is experienced with sugar.

Eat whole grain starches: Blood-sugar levels rise slowly and steadily for up to 4 hours. Insulin is released in small steady amounts from the pancreas, resulting in even blood-sugar levels and no dramatic drop in blood sugar as is seen with sugar or refined grains.

Eating extra dietary carbohydrate (starches and sugars) will raise Serotonin, which makes you feel calm and relaxed. So you can see how the usual combination of sugar and fat (many desserts) set you up to feel calm and content, and can easily set up cravings for additional desserts because you want that inner state of calm and contentment.

Stress is also a common reason given for overeating or emotional eating. Two out of three people eat more under stress. Plus, we don't usually overeat vegetables when we're stressed. You can make small changes over time to improve eating habits. Do your best to choose foods rich in nutrients when you are under stress. For example: vegetables, fruits, whole grains, lean protein, and healthy fats in moderation. Limit sugar, unhealthy fat, caffeine, and alcohol.

When loneliness or stress increase, this leads to an increase in Cortisol, which leads to deposits of abdominal fat and makes it more difficult to lose weight or keep it off.

Do you sleep enough? 7-9 hours of sleep is vital to your health. There is a strong link between the amount of sleep people get and their risk of becoming overweight. Sleep deprivation decreases Leptin, a blood protein that suppresses appetite, and increases Ghrelin, a substance that makes people want to eat. After a night of sleep deprivation, people typically consume 10 percent more calories!

If you feel inferior, have the "blues", think you need to find something or want a reward, this leads to the increase of Dopamine, which will lead to an increase in desire for food, and an increase in attention to searching out enjoyable eating experiences or rewarding actions.

Calming and positive thoughts lead to an increase in Serotonin, which lowers your desire for food, and increases your satisfaction, all of which helps control your temper, improve your sleep, while balancing sexual urges, and enhancing your memory.

When you eat favorite food this will increase Endorphins, which may also lead to an increase in your eating speed, which causes you to eat more.

Endorphins (the body's natural Opiates which give a "high") when they are low, this leads to an increase of the urge to get relief or pleasure, desire for junk foods, excess exercise, or alcohol.

Exercise naturally raises Endorphins and control NPY 9neuropeptide Y) which lowers anxiety and carbohydrate cravings and increases feelings of contentment.

After a person exercises, abnormal Cortisol levels lower, Dopamine lowers (arousal hormone), and Norepinephrine lower, which leads to appetite suppression and mood stability and you feel better.

APPENDIX C

Specific cravings and addictions

Sugar:
- Need for brain fuel or energy
- Need for body fuel or energy
- Deficiency of amino acids or protein
- Presence of infection or yeast in the body. Bacteria, yeast, viruses, parasites, cancer cells thrive on sugar

Alcohol:
- Need for brain fuel or energy
- Need for body fuel or energy
- Hypoglycemia – poor sugar metabolism and protein deficiency
- Presence of yeast in the body – As alcohol is fermented, yeast or candida in the body can cause you to crave alcohol in order to feed the yeast. This is especially true with beer and wine.

Bread, cereal, pasta:
- Need for brain and body fuel
- Unbalanced blood sugar
- Presence of infection or yeast in the body

Salt:
- Need for minerals for supporting the adrenal glands in producing energy
- Dehydration or need for water – The body craves salt to help retain water.

Cheese:
- Need for EFA's (essential fatty acids) for brain power
- Need for proteins/amino acids for proper neurotransmission for balanced brain chemistry
- Need protein/amino acids for muscle fuel

Spicy or highly seasoned food:
- Need for nutrients, especially vitamins and minerals

- Need for Zinc – When deficient, it can lead to impaired sense of taste and smell. Some people require strong tasting food because they don't taste anything otherwise.

Ice:
- Need for Iron – Person may be Anemic.
- Need for folic acid, B6, or B12

Acid or sour food:
- Body is full of toxins

Fish and shrimp:
- Iodine deficiency
- Hypothyroidism

Licorice:
- Salt and/or water deficiency (Licorice increases retention of water therefore leading to High Blood Pressure)

Dirt or clay:
- Need for minerals or other nutrients – People with the eating disorder, pica, crave non-food substances. The body is looking for nutrition from dirt, clay, soap, paint chips, cigarette ashes, or broken crockery. Serious mineral deficiencies, as well as metal toxicity can lead to this disorder.

APPENDIX D

If you crave…What you really need…Healthy alternatives!

Chocolate – (Magnesium) Raw nuts and seeds, legumes, fruits

Sweets – (Chromium) Broccoli, grapes, cheese, dried beans, chicken

Sweets – (Carbon) Fresh Fruit

Sweets – (Phosphorus) Chicken, beef, liver, poultry, fish, eggs, dairy, nuts, legumes, grains

Sweets – (Sulfur) Cranberries, horseradish, cruciferous vegetables, kale, cabbage

Sweets – (Tryptophan) Cheese, liver, lamb, raisins, sweet potatoes, spinach

Bread, Toast – (Nitrogen) High protein foods: fish, meat, nuts, beans

Oily snacks, Fatty foods – (Calcium) Mustard and turnip greens, broccoli, kale, legumes, cheese, sesame

Coffee or Tea – (Phosphorus) Chicken, beef, liver, poultry, fish, eggs, dairy, nuts, legumes

Coffee and Tea – (Sulfur) Egg yolks, red peppers, muscle protein, garlic, onion, cruciferous vegetables

Coffee and Tea – (NaCl-Salt) Sea salt, apple cider vinegar (on salad)

Coffee and Tea – (Iron) Meat, fish and poultry, seaweed, greens, black cherries

Alcohol, recreational drugs – (Protein) Meat, poultry, seafood, dairy, nuts

Alcohol, recreational drugs – (Avenin) Granola, oatmeal

Alcohol, recreational drugs – (Calcium) Mustard and turnip greens, broccoli, kale, legumes, cheese, sesame

Alcohol, recreational drugs –
(Glutamine) Supplement glutamine powder for withdrawal, raw cabbage juice

Alcohol, recreational drugs –
(Potassium) Sun-dried black olives, potato peel broth, seaweed, bitter greens

Chewing ice – (Iron) Meat, fish, poultry, seaweed, greens, black cherries

Burned food – (Carbon) Fresh fruits

Soda and other carbonated drinks –
(Calcium) Mustard and turnip greens, broccoli, kale, legumes, cheese, sesame

Salty foods – (Chloride) Raw goat milk, fish, unrefined sea salt

Acid foods – (Magnesium) Raw nuts and seeds, legumes, fruits

Liquids rather than solids – (Water) Flavor water with lemon or lime. You need 8-10 glasses per day.

Solids rather than liquids – (Water) You are dehydrated Flavor water with lemon or lime and drink 8-10 glasses per day

Cool drinks – (Manganese) Walnuts, almonds, pecans, pineapple, blueberries

Pre-menstrual craving – (Zinc) Red meats (especially organ), seafood, leafy vegetables, root vegetables

General Overeating – (Silicon) Nuts, seeds, avoid refined starches

General Overeating – (Tryptophan) Cheese, liver, lamb, raisins, sweet potato, spinach

General Overeating – (Tyrosine) Vitamin C supplements or orange, green, red fruits and vegetables

Lack of appetite – (Vitamin B1) Nuts, seeds, beans, liver and other organ meats

Lack of appetite – (Vitamin B3) Tuna, halibut, beef, chicken, turkey, pork, seeds and legumes

Lack of appetite – (Manganese) Walnuts, almonds, pecans, pineapple, blueberries

Lack of appetite – (Chloride) Raw goat milk, unrefined sea salt

Tobacco – (Silicon) Nuts, seeds, avoid refined starches

Tobacco – (Tyrosine) Vitamin C supplements or orange, green, and red fruits and vegetables

APPENDIX E

The Glycemic Index (GI)
The best ways to keep insulin and blood sugar levels low is to eat carbohydrates that rank low on the glycemic index. This index shows the rate at which carbohydrates break down as sugar or glucose in the bloodstream. Foods that are high-glycemic index release glucose into the bloodstream quickly causing a rapid rise in blood sugar and a subsequent rise in insulin. Low-glycemic foods usually contain more fiber and release glucose into the bloodstream at a slower rate.

HIGH 70 percent and up
MODERATE 40 percent – 69 percent
LOW 39 percent and below

Rapid Inducers of Insulin
GI - 100 percent or greater
Puffed Rice
Corn Flakes
Beer

Puffed Wheat
French Baguette
Instant White Rice
Jelly Beans
Rice Krispies
Rice Chex
Millet
Cheerios
Glucose
White Bread
Bagel
Whole Wheat Bread

GI 90 percent – 99 percent
Raisins
Grapenuts
Carrots
Parsnips
Barley (whole meal)
Nutri-grain (Kellogg)
Watermelon
Muesli
Shredded Wheat
Apricots
Corn Chips

GI 80 percent – 89 percent
Rolled Oats
Oat Bran
Honey
White Rice (long grain)
Brown Rice
White Potato
Orange Juice
Corn
Rye (whole meal)
Ripe Banana
Mango
Papaya
Bran Chex

GI 79 percent – 70 percent
Kidney Beans
Wheat
Oatmeal
Chocolate
Buckwheat
Oatmeal Cookies
Waffles
Kiwi
Fruit Cocktail (Del Monte)

Moderate Inducers of Insulin
GI 60 percent – 69 percent
Spaghetti (white & whole wheat)
Pinto Beans
Macaroni
Rye (pumpernickel)
Full fat Ice Cream
Pizza
Couscous
Wheat Kernels
Beets
Apple Juice
Applesauce
Popcorn

GI 50 percent – 59 percent
Potato Chips
Barley
Green Banana
Lactose
Peas (frozen)
Par Broiled Rice (uncle bens)
Sucrose
Yam
Custard
Dried White Beans

GI 40 percent – 49 percent
Sweet Potato
Navy Beans
Peas (dried)
Lima Beans
Apples
Baked Beans
Butter Beans
Rye (whole grain)

Reduced Insulin Secretion
GI 30 percent – 39 percent
Pears
Tomato Soup
Black-eyed Peas
Chickpeas
Milk (skim)
Milk (whole)
Yogurt (low fat)
All-Bran

GI 20 percent – 29 percent
Lentils
Fructose
Plums
Dried Peas
Peaches

Grapefruit
Cherries

GI 10 percent – 19 percent
Soybeans
Peanuts

These numbers vary by 10-15 percent depending on the standards used. You can look them up to be more accurate. The Glycemic Index does not mean that the food is bad or good for you; it simply states the rate at which the body breaks down the food.

APPENDIX F

Carbohydrates are necessary to your health, because every cell in your body uses them for energy. Your brain can only use carbohydrates for energy. Over-consumption of sugar, high-fructose corn syrup, and other highly refined carbohydrates has been associated with a higher incidence of diabetes, cardiovascular disease, and even breast cancer. Eating refined carbs can, over time, result in almost uncontrollable sugar cravings.
Complex carbohydrates are high-fiber foods, which improve your digestion. They help stabilize the blood sugar, keep your energy at an even level, and help you feel satisfied longer after your meal.
In contrast, sugar and other simple carbohydrates can alter your mood, lead to cravings and compulsive eating, cause wide swings in your blood sugar levels, and cause weight gain in most people. In addition, a high consumption of sugar can lead to uncomfortable withdrawal symptoms when you finally

decide to improve your diet and forgo
the sweets.

Healthy Complex Carbohydrates
Spinach
Turnip greens
Lettuce
Watercress
Zucchini
Asparagus
Artichokes
Okra
Cabbage
Celery
Cucumbers
Dill pickles
Broccoli
Brussels sprouts
Whole barley
Buckwheat
Oat bran
Oatmeal
Oat bran
Wild rice
Brown rice
Multi-grain bread

Pinto beans
Yogurt
Navy beans
Cauliflower
Grapefruit
Apples
Yams

Simple Carbohydrates
Table Sugar
Corn Syrup
Fruit Juice
Candy
Cake
White Bread
White Pasta
Soda
White Baked Goods
Most Packaged Cereal

If you are trying to eliminate simple sugars and carbohydrates from your diet, but you don't want to refer to this list all the time, here are some suggestions:

Read the Labels. If the label lists sugar, sucrose, fructose, corn syrup, white or "wheat", they contain simple carbohydrates. If these ingredients are at the top of the list, they may contain mostly simple carbohydrates, and little else. They should be avoided.

APPENDIX G

Recommendations if you have food cravings

Variety – Do not get in rut of eating the same things over and over. Eat a variety of colors and different foods.

Don't skip meals – Preferably eat 3 meals with snacks included between meals. Don't go longer than 4 hours between meals. Prolonged bouts of not eating results in low blood sugar and we compensate by overeating later.

Don't skip breakfast – Giving your body a stable supply of blood sugar first thing in the morning will attenuate hunger and reduce chance of overeating later in the day.

Combine Protein/fat or Carbs/fat at each meal or snack – Combining macronutrients will provide a steady supply of blood sugar and keep you full longer without unbalanced insulin levels

Drink Water – Our body often confuses hunger with thirst (dehydration). Drink a glass before your meal and re-evaluate how hungry you are.

Eat a small amount of the food you are craving – By trying to cut out a particular craved food "cold turkey", it can increase the desire to consume it and lead to over-indulging on it later.

*Sniff Mint – Study shows that sniffing peppermint throughout the day disrupts the craving.

*Tap your forehead – Scientific theory says when a craving comes on, place your 5 fingers on your forehead and tap each finger at intervals while looking up at them. The craving will have disappeared.

System for eliminating food cravings

- 8 ounces of water immediately when you begin to crave any food
- No starches with the evening meal (only protein, vegetables and healthy fats)
- Sparkling water with mint gum after dinner, every night

- Supplementation with mult-vitamin/mineral every day
- Elimination of appetite stimulating artificial sweeteners (sucralose/splenda, acesulfame potassium, aspartame, NutraSweet). Only exceptions are the trace amounts in gum
- Jumping jacks, body weight pushups or squats for 2 minutes when you begin to crave any food.

BIBLIOGRAPHY

http://www.livingwhole.com
http://www.scicn.com
http://www.naturalhealthtechniques.com
http://www.balancedweightmanagement.com
Food & Mood; Elizabeth Somer, M.A., R.D.